# PANCREAS TRANSPLANT DIET

## A Comprehensive Guide To Nutritional Support, Surgery Recovery And Controlling Blood Sugar Level

## DR LUCAS KAYCE

# DISCLAIMER

This book about illness and nutrition is not meant to replace expert medical advice, diagnosis, or treatment; rather, it is meant purely for informational reasons. This book's content is founded on broad concepts and recommendations for managing diseases and nutrition.

Before adopting any major dietary or lifestyle changes, readers are recommended to speak with a qualified healthcare provider, such as a licensed physician or registered dietitian, especially if they have pre-existing medical concerns. Everybody has different health demands, so what works for one person might not work for another.

The use of the information provided in this book may have unfavorable repercussions or consequences, for which the author and publisher disclaim all liability. No disease is meant to be identified, treated, cured, or prevented by the information provided.

The book may include contain references to medical literature or research findings; however readers are urged to independently confirm this material and contact reliable sources.

It is important to remember that the fields of nutrition and medicine are always changing, and that new findings could have an impact on the advice offered in this book. As a result, readers are urged to keep up with the most recent advancements in healthcare and, when in doubt, seek professional counsel.

By reading this book, readers agree that they are in charge of their own health decisions and release the author and publisher from any liability arising from the use of the material in the book, whether direct or indirect.

# TABLE OF CONTENTS

# ABOUT THE BOOK

"Pancreas Transplant Diet," a detailed and insightful guide to post-transplant care through a specialized diet, is an invaluable resource for anyone who has had a pancreas transplant. This book is significant because it offers a thorough overview of pancreas transplants, illuminating the subtleties of post-transplant care and the critical role nutrition plays in the healing process.

The book set the stage by explaining to readers the complexities of pancreatic transplants and stressing the importance of a comprehensive approach to treatment. The book then dives into the fundamentals of a diet that is healthy for the pancreas, explaining the importance of a balanced diet and the necessary nutrients. This comprehensive investigation also covers the management of drugs and how they interact with nutrition, providing doable tactics to balance these two important facets of life after transplantation.

The comprehensive Pancreas Transplant Diet Plan, which gives readers useful tools for meal planning, suggested food groups, and portion control, is one of the book's best aspects. The book also covers special aspects including managing blood sugar, digestive problems, and adjusting to weight fluctuations, indicating a thorough comprehension of the particular difficulties faced by recipients of pancreatic transplants.

The book expands on dietary considerations by highlighting lifestyle elements that are crucial for a successful transplant, including consistent exercise, stress reduction, and enough sleep.

A useful component is added with helpful advice on interacting with people and dining out, which gives readers ways to express dietary requirements and make decisions in a variety of contexts.

The book on tracking and modifying food, promoting routine examinations, and offering guidance on identifying indicators of nutritional inadequacies all demonstrate its dedication to continuing care. The nutritional guidelines become more approachable and tasty with the addition of a range of dishes for a pancreas-healthy way of living.

"Pancreas Transplant Diet" is an invaluable tool that provides a comprehensive approach to life after transplantation, going beyond standard medical advice. It equips readers with information and useful tactics so that those facing the difficulties of pancreatic transplants can maximize their recuperation by using a customized and educated dietary approach.

# CHAPTER ONE

## PANCREAS TRANSPLANT DIET OVERVIEW

## THE VALUE OF A CUSTOMIZED DIET FOLLOWING A PANCREAS TRANSPLANT

It is impossible to exaggerate the importance of a particular diet after a pancreas transplant since it is crucial to the overall outcome of the procedure. A complicated medical surgery known as a pancreatic transplant is used to replace a failing or non-functioning pancreas, usually in patients who have diabetes. In addition to restoring insulin production, this life-changing procedure calls for extensive lifestyle modifications, such as a customized nutrition plan.

## KNOWING ABOUT TRANSPLANTS OF THE PANCREAS

A healthy pancreas from a deceased donor is surgically transplanted into a recipient who lacks or has a malfunctioning pancreatic. For those with type 1 diabetes or serious diabetes-related problems, the operation is frequently advised. Restoring normal insulin production is the goal to reduce the requirement for exogenous insulin delivery. Through this complex surgical procedure, patients can potentially regain control over their blood sugar levels and enhance their overall quality of life.

## A SYNOPSIS OF PANCREATIC TRANSPLANTS

Producing insulin and digestive enzymes, the pancreas is an essential organ in the endocrine and digestive systems. Serious health problems can arise when the pancreas is not functioning at its best, especially in those who have diabetes.

Thus, a pancreatic transplant becomes a feasible solution to deal with these problems. To reduce the chance of rejection, donors and recipients are carefully matched during the transplantation process. The actual operation is a difficult procedure that requires the knowledge of a highly qualified surgical team.

# AFTER-TRANSPLANT CARE AND THINGS TO THINK ABOUT

Even more crucial than the actual surgery is the time after a pancreatic transplant. To minimize difficulties and guarantee that the recipient's body takes the new organ, post-transplant care entails a multimodal approach. Post-transplant care must include close observation, immunosuppressive drugs, and following physician recommendations. Recipients should also be alert for any indications of rejection or infection, emphasizing the value of routine check-ups and consultation with medical experts.

## DIET'S FUNCTION IN THE RECUPERATION OF TRANSPLANTS

After a pancreas transplant, diet is vitally important to overall healing. To control blood sugar levels, aid in the healing process, and improve the functioning of the transplanted organ, a particular diet is frequently advised. Restrictions on specific foods may be part of nutritional guidelines to reduce the risk of consequences and encourage a healthy lifestyle. Furthermore, the dietary guidelines are customized to meet the specific requirements of the transplant recipient, taking into account their age, general health, and any pre-existing medical issues.

For those struggling with issues associated with diabetes, a pancreas transplant is a life-changing procedure. The road to recovery, however, goes beyond the operation, highlighting the critical significance that a particular diet plays in guaranteeing the transplant's success. Recipients hoping for more than simply a new organ must comprehend the complexities of pancreas transplants, the importance of post-transplant care, and customized dietary recommendations.

# CHAPTER TWO

## ESSENTIALS OF A DIET FOR PANCREAS HEALTH

## NUTRITIONAL NEEDS FOLLOWING TRANSPLANT

Following pancreatic transplant surgery, eating a pancreas-healthy diet becomes essential to the procedure's overall success. The process of transplantation not only modifies the pancreatic physiological dynamics but also places particular dietary demands on the body of the recipient. Restoring insulin production and regulation is important, and it necessitates paying close attention to nutritional consumption.

Following a transplant, patients should concentrate on eating a balanced diet that promotes recovery and ensures the transplanted pancreas operates at its best. Consuming enough protein is crucial for supporting tissue regeneration and repair while the body heals from the surgery.

Furthermore, since micronutrients like vitamins and minerals are essential to many metabolic processes that are critical to general health, it is imperative to pay close attention to these nutrients.

The metabolism and absorption of nutrients can be impacted by the immunosuppressive drugs that are frequently administered after transplantation to prevent rejection. As such, it's critical to closely monitor nutrient levels and modify the diet as needed. It is advised to work with a medical professional or a trained dietitian to customize the diet to each person's needs and make sure that the nutritional requirements are satisfied after transplant.

## THE VALUE OF A WELL-BALANCED DIET

For people who have had pancreas transplants or not, eating a healthy, balanced diet is essential since it has a direct impact on general health and well-being. A balanced diet is especially important for recipients of pancreas transplants since they require good organ function and immune system support.

A well-balanced diet helps the body adjust to the changes brought about by the transplant and helps prevent problems.

The essential macronutrients—carbohydrates, proteins, and fats—are provided in the right amounts by a balanced diet. Proteins help maintain and repair tissue, carbohydrates are essential for energy production, and healthy fats maintain and promote cellular structure and function. Furthermore, fiber—which can be found in fruits, vegetables, and whole grains—supports healthy digestion and aids in blood sugar regulation, which is especially important for pancreatic health.

In addition, eating a diet high in fruits and vegetables that are high in antioxidants helps fight oxidative stress, which is important for preserving cellular integrity and reducing inflammation.

Maintaining proper hydration is crucial for supporting multiple body processes, such as digestion and nutrition transportation. All things considered, maintaining the longevity and ideal function of the transplanted pancreas is mostly dependent on eating a balanced diet.

## NUTRITIONAL RECOMMENDATIONS FOR OPTIMAL PANCREATIC FUNCTION

Dietary guidelines for pancreatic optimization entail a multifaceted approach that considers a range of nutritional factors. First and foremost, entire, nutrient-dense foods including fruits, vegetables, whole grains, lean meats, and healthy fats are recommended for consumption. These foods support general metabolic health in addition to offering vital nutrients.

It's critical to watch and control how much carbohydrates you eat, especially if you have received a pancreas transplant. Selecting complex carbs rather than simple sugars facilitates efficient blood glucose regulation.

Controlling portion sizes and eating regularly throughout the day can help stabilize blood sugar levels and avoid crashes and surges that could put undue stress on the pancreatic transplant.

Including omega-3 fatty acids—which are present in walnuts, flaxseeds, and fatty fish—can enhance pancreas function and have anti-inflammatory properties. It is advised to limit intake of saturated and trans fats because high intake might aggravate inflammation and impair normal organ function.

Maintaining an appropriate fluid intake is important for pancreatic health, thus people should strive to stay hydrated. Water helps the transplanted pancreas work properly by promoting healthy digestion, nutrient absorption, and overall cellular function.

It is crucial to regularly test blood levels, particularly glucose and lipid profiles, to adjust the dietary strategy and make sure that the nutritional recommendations are promoting pancreatic function. Working along with medical specialists, such as dietitians and transplant specialists, is essential to customizing dietary advice to each patient's needs and ensuring the pancreas transplant has long-term success.

# CHAPTER THREE

## TAKING CARE OF DRUG AND FOOD INTERACTIONS

### SYNOPSIS OF DRUGS USED IN TRANSPLANTATION

When it comes to the postoperative treatment of patients who have had organ transplants, transplant drugs are essential.

The main goal of these drugs is to weaken the immune system of the recipient so that the newly transplanted organ won't be attacked and rejected. In this situation, immunosuppressants such as tacrolimus, cyclosporine, mycophenolate mofetil, and corticosteroids are often recommended drugs.

Each of these medications targets distinct immune system pathways to preserve the precarious equilibrium between limiting adverse effects and avoiding rejection.

# RELATIONSHIPS BETWEEN FOOD AND MEDICINE

The complex interaction between food and medicine can have a big effect on how well a patient responds to treatment as a whole. Dietary concerns are important when it comes to transplant drugs because of possible interactions that can change the efficacy, metabolism, or absorption of the drug. For example, certain meals may interfere with the way immunosuppressive medications are absorbed, causing variations in blood levels. For instance, it is well known that grapefruit juice can disrupt the way that certain drugs are metabolized, leading to an increase in their bloodstream levels and possible side effects. To guarantee the best possible performance of their prescription medications, transplant recipients must be informed of such interactions.

Furthermore, food ingredients like vitamin K may interact with anticoagulant drugs like warfarin. To avoid variations in the anticoagulant's efficacy, vitamin

K-containing foods must be consumed consistently. However, due to possible adverse effects, some drugs may require special dietary restrictions. For example, corticosteroids can cause a loss of bone density, thus people need to concentrate on meals and supplements high in calcium.

## TECHNIQUES FOR HARMONIZING MEDICINE AND DIET

Finding a balance between medicine and diet is a complex process that calls for an all-encompassing strategy. To create a customized strategy that meets each patient's specific needs, healthcare professionals—including transplant specialists, nutritionists, and pharmacists—must communicate with one another. A more stable treatment plan can be achieved by making dietary alterations in addition to routinely monitoring drug levels and potential adverse effects.

Transplant recipients need education to appropriately manage their drug regimen and dietary issues. Patients need to be informed about the value of making consistent food and drug choices. People can make more educated decisions about their daily routines when they are aware of the unique requirements of their prescriptions, such as whether or not to take them with food.

Adopting lifestyle changes, such as eating a balanced diet, working out frequently, and abstaining from potentially dangerous substances like tobacco or excessive alcohol, enhances the overall success of transplantation. These lifestyle decisions can improve general health, medication metabolism, and the immune system.

The effectiveness of organ transplantation depends on the management of food and pharmaceutical combinations. The general health and lifespan of transplant patients are influenced by a thorough understanding of transplant drugs, awareness of possible drug-food interactions, and adoption of techniques to balance medication and diet.

# CHAPTER FOUR

## THE DIET PLAN FOR PANCREAS TRANSPLANTS

## PLANNING MEALS FOR PATIENTS RECEIVING PANCREAS TRANSPLANTS

Following pancreas transplant surgery, recipients must follow a nutritious, well-balanced diet plan to promote their general health and preserve the function of the freshly transplanted organ.

To ensure that recipients of transplants obtain the nutrients they require without endangering the health of the pancreatic graft, meal planning is essential.

Keeping blood sugar levels steady is one of the important factors pancreas transplant recipients must take into account while planning their meals. Insulin is produced by the pancreas, and following transplantation, the host and the transplanted organ share responsibility for controlling blood glucose levels.

Consequently, to prevent unexpected spikes or falls in blood sugar, recipients are frequently encouraged to consume regular, balanced meals throughout the day.

## SUGGESTED FOOD GROUPS AND AMOUNTS

For pancreas transplant recipients, a well-rounded diet usually consists of a range of nutrient-dense foods from various food categories. A balanced diet that includes a variety of fruits, vegetables, whole grains, lean meats, and healthy fats guarantees that all the important vitamins and minerals are consumed. Whole grains, fruits, and vegetables are examples of foods high in fiber that are essential for preserving digestive health and controlling blood sugar levels.

Another essential element that helps with tissue upkeep and healing is protein. It's common advice to eat lean protein sources including fish, fowl, tofu, and lentils. Keeping an eye on portion sizes is crucial since consuming too many calories can lead to weight gain and other problems.

Recipients receiving pancreas transplants should avoid processed foods, sugary snacks, and high-fat foods as much as possible. To control blood pressure and avoid fluid retention—which can be especially problematic after a transplant—it is essential to monitor sodium intake.

## SAMPLE RECIPES AND MEAL PLANS

For pancreas transplant recipients, maintaining a balanced diet requires developing varied and tasty meal plans. A modest handful of almonds, a portion of fresh fruit, and whole-grain cereal with low-fat milk may be a sample breakfast. A vibrant salad full of leafy greens, lean protein, and different vegetables is a healthy choice for lunch. Steamed veggies, brown rice, quinoa, and grilled fish or chicken might be the meal.

Selecting healthy snacks is important. Some ideas are Greek yogurt, hummus-topped raw veggies, or a tiny bowl of mixed almonds. It's critical to maintain proper hydration throughout the day by consuming enough water.

Simple recipes that use fresh ingredients and minimal processed or high-sugar additives are popular among recipients of pancreatic transplants. Healthy and tasty meals can be found in stir-fries with a variety of veggies and lean protein, oven-baked fish flavored with herbs, and quinoa bowls topped with vibrant vegetables.

The food plan for pancreatic transplantation prioritizes moderation, diversity, and balance. Recipients can enjoy a fulfilling and savory dining experience while helping to ensure the long-term success of their transplant by embracing a varied range of nutrient-rich foods and being mindful of portion sizes.

# CHAPTER FIVE

## PARTICULAR ATTENTION TO RECIPIENTS OF PANCREAS TRANSPLANTS

### CONTROLLING BLOOD SUGAR LEVELS

Controlling blood sugar levels is an essential part of caring for recipients of pancreatic transplants because problems can be avoided by maintaining ideal glycemic control. It is anticipated that the transplanted pancreas will generate insulin, enabling recipients to better control their blood glucose levels. Recipients must, however, periodically check their blood sugar, take their medications as directed, and modify their lifestyle as needed. It is essential to work closely with healthcare providers to create a customized treatment plan that takes into account each patient's unique dietary and insulin requirements.

### HANDLING DIGESTIVE PROBLEMS

Managing Digestive Problems is another important factor for recipients of pancreatic transplants. The digestive system is essential for absorbing nutrients, and after transplantation, changes in its operation may take place. Gastrointestinal problems like gas, bloating, or changes in bowel habits may affect some recipients. These problems may be related to immunological responses, medicines, or the body's adjustment to the new organ. It takes a multidisciplinary team of transplant doctors, dietitians, and gastroenterologists to treat and manage digestive issues and make sure recipients can continue to eat a healthy, balanced diet.

## MANAGING WEIGHT SHIFTS

One of the inevitable aspects of the post-pancreas transplant experience is adjusting to weight changes. Patients may have fluctuations in their weight for a variety of reasons, such as modifications to their food, adverse effects from medication, and changes in their metabolism. While some individuals may struggle to maintain or gain weight, others may experience weight increase. Combining dietary changes, frequent exercise, and continuing medical supervision are all part of a comprehensive weight-management strategy. This takes into account each recipient's unique demands and preferences while ensuring that they reach and maintain a weight that is appropriate for their general health.

Recipients of pancreatic transplants have unique needs that go beyond the actual surgical process. Handling Digestive Problems, Managing Blood Sugar Levels, and Adjusting to Weight Changes are all essential parts of the comprehensive care needed for the best possible results after transplantation. To fully address these factors and customize interventions to each recipient's needs, recipients and medical experts must work together to improve the overall quality of life for pancreas transplant recipients.

..

# CHAPTER SIX

## LIFESTYLE ELEMENTS FOR A SUCCESSFUL TRANSPLANT

### REGULAR EXERCISE IS CRUCIAL

Frequent exercise is an essential part of a transplant patient's lifestyle. Frequent physical activity is essential for overall health and is particularly critical for the outcome of a transplant procedure. Exercise fortifies the immune system, strengthens the heart, and increases the body's capacity to withstand the stress of organ transplantation. Furthermore, it's critical to regularly exercise to maintain a healthy weight because obesity raises the chance of problems after transplantation. Improved circulation is another benefit of exercise for the healthy operation of the transplanted organ.

### TECHNIQUES FOR STRESS MANAGEMENT

Techniques for managing stress are just as crucial for a transplant to be successful. The way transplant recipients feel emotionally and psychologically can have a big influence on how well the surgery goes. Prolonged stress can have a deleterious impact on one's general health and immune system, which may cause issues during the post-transplant phase. Using stress-reduction strategies like therapy, mindfulness, or meditation can lessen the psychological toll that organ transplantation takes. Establishing a positive outlook and building a support network are essential components of stress management that can facilitate a quicker healing process.

## SLEEPING ENOUGH

Getting enough sleep is essential to the healing process after a transplant. The body's ability to mend itself and maintain general health depends heavily on sleep. Patients undergoing transplants may find it difficult to get a good night's sleep because of the anxiety associated with the surgery, their medications, or schedule changes. To make sure transplant recipients get the rest they need, it's critical to set up a regular sleep regimen and create a cozy sleep environment. Immune system performance is strongly correlated with sleep quality, and a well-rested body is better able to withstand the demands of organ donation. Healthcare providers frequently stress how crucial it is to prioritize sleep as part of an all-encompassing post-transplant care plan.

A healthy lifestyle that includes regular exercise, stress reduction practices, and enough sleep all helps organ transplant recipients recover. These components help the mental and emotional aspects of the transplant journey in addition to enhancing physical well-being. Transplant recipients can have an overall improvement in quality of life and a more effective recovery process if a holistic approach to post-transplant care is implemented, taking into account certain lifestyle aspects.

# CHAPTER SEVEN

## COMMUNICATING DIETARY NEEDS

## MANAGING SOCIAL SITUATIONS

When interacting with others in social settings and when dining out, it's critical to communicate your dietary requirements. To guarantee a satisfying eating experience, it is essential to communicate dietary restrictions and preferences clearly and effectively. It is polite to let the host or restaurant personnel know in advance if you have any special dietary needs when you are invited to a party or restaurant. This enables them to take your demands into account and make appropriate plans. Expressing your dietary demands, whether because of personal preferences, religious convictions, or allergies, promotes inclusivity and guarantees that everyone may eat with ease.

It's critical to be precise and unambiguous when expressing dietary requirements, including any restrictions or preferences.

Giving hosts and restaurant employees comprehensive information enables them to make well-informed choices on the menu and meal preparation. Additionally, it helps to show your appreciation for any accommodations made on your behalf. This will assist in building goodwill and facilitate more easy interactions in the future.

## MAKING KNOWLEDGEABLE DECISIONS AT RESTAURANTS

Making educated decisions is essential to preserving a happy and healthful dining experience in restaurants. Making decisions that support one's nutritional objectives can be facilitated by taking the time to browse the menu and enquire about ingredients or preparation techniques. These days, a lot of restaurants provide a range of options, such as gluten-free, vegetarian, vegan, and other dietary-specific foods. Being proactive in obtaining menu information might enable people to choose meals that satisfy their taste preferences in addition to meeting their nutritional needs.

It helps to be well-prepared while making decisions at restaurants. Learning popular terminology from the menu, like sautéed, steamed, and grilled, might help one become more aware of healthy cooking techniques. Furthermore, the culinary staff frequently accommodates requests for substitutes or alterations, enabling patrons to tailor their meals to better meet their dietary requirements.

## ENJOYING SPECIAL OCCASIONS WITHOUT PUTTING YOUR DIET AT RISK

It takes careful planning to enjoy special occasions without sacrificing one's diet. Even while it's tempting to overindulge during celebrations, there are ways to enjoy special occasions without going too far from one's nutritional objectives.

Planning might be useful in instances where options that fit one's diet may be restricted. One way to avoid overindulging is to eat a healthy meal before going to an event. Furthermore, bringing a meal that complies with individual dietary requirements guarantees that there will be something for everyone, adding to the enjoyment of the event for all guests.

It is possible to enjoy special occasions without sacrificing one's diet, which is an essential component of social life. Preparing beforehand guarantees guilt-free celebrations, whether it's consuming a balanced lunch before the occasion or bringing food that complies with personal dietary preferences. It's important to strike a balance between overindulgence and strict dietary guidelines so that people can enjoy the holidays without sacrificing their health and well-being.

Navigating social situations and dining out with specific dietary restrictions requires efficient communication, smart planning, and informed decision-making. Through understanding these ideas, people can celebrate and form deep friendships without sacrificing their nutritional objectives.

# CHAPTER EIGHT

## KEEPING AN EYE ON AND MODIFYING THE DIET

### FREQUENT EXAMINATIONS AND EVALUATIONS

Monitoring and modifying one's diet to maintain optimal health and well-being requires regular check-ups and assessments. These routine exams, performed by medical professionals, are preventative steps to find any possible problems or imbalances in a person's nutritional state. During these examinations, several health markers, such as blood pressure, cholesterol, and body mass index (BMI), are usually thoroughly assessed. To identify dietary excesses or deficiencies, medical professionals may also use blood tests to measure the amounts of particular nutrients.

The number of these examinations may differ depending on your age, general health, and any current medical issues. People with particular nutritional preferences or chronic conditions, for example, might require more frequent monitoring to meet their special demands. Frequent examinations not only aid in the identification of nutritional imbalances but also give medical practitioners the chance to make individualized dietary and lifestyle suggestions.

## IDENTIFYING NUTRITIONAL DEFICIENCIES' SIGNS

Maintaining a balanced and healthful diet requires being able to recognize the warning symptoms of nutritional deficits. When the body is deficient in certain nutrients, it might cause certain symptoms that indicate the need to make dietary changes. For instance, weakness, exhaustion, and a prolonged lack of energy could be signs of an iron or vitamin B12 deficiency. Dryness or atypical coloring on the skin may indicate a deficiency in vitamins A, C, or E.

Other indicators of nutritional abnormalities include sluggish wound healing, brittle nails, and hair loss. Inadequate consumption of specific vitamins and minerals may also be associated with cognitive symptoms such as trouble focusing, memory problems, or mood swings. People must be aware of these symptoms and seek the advice and appropriate examination of healthcare professionals.

## ADJUSTING THE DIET AS NECESSARY

Dietary modifications are a dynamic and continuing process that is made in response to specific health demands and nutritional inadequacies. Dietary changes are required to address particular shortages or excesses after examinations reveal evidence of nutritional imbalances. Dietary changes may include adding more nutrient-dense items to the diet, such as whole grains, fruits, vegetables, and lean meats.

Under the supervision of medical professionals, supplementation may be advised in cases of deficiency. It is crucial to remember that to guarantee long-term adherence, dietary adjustments should be customized to individual tastes, cultural concerns, and lifestyle circumstances.

Maintaining a well-balanced and nutritionally appropriate diet requires regular discussion with healthcare practitioners, nutritionists, or dietitians to track progress, make necessary adjustments, and receive continuous support.

# CHAPTER NINE

BREAKFAST IDEAS AND RECIPES

## PANCREAS-HEALTHY LIFESTYLE

Having a pancreas-healthy breakfast is essential to sustaining steady blood sugar levels all day. Choosing whole grains, like quinoa or oats, is an excellent supply of fiber that promotes healthy digestion and reduces blood sugar increases. Try adding some fresh fruit, such as apples or berries, as they naturally sweeten food without raising blood sugar levels too much. Another great option is eggs, which have enough protein to keep you feeling content and full.

Smoothies consisting of low-sugar fruits, veggies, and a protein source, like almond butter or Greek yogurt, provide a handy and wholesome choice. Pay attention to added sugars and use natural sweeteners sparingly, such as honey or maple syrup.

A balanced breakfast can also benefit from the addition of healthy fats like those found in almonds or avocados, which can help to maintain energy levels throughout the morning.

## RECIPES FOR LUNCH AND DINNER

Lean protein sources, such as grilled chicken, turkey, or fish, are easier on the pancreas and are a great choice for pancreas-healthy lunches and dinners. A range of vital nutrients is ensured by including a diversity of colored vegetables, and choosing non-starchy veggies such as leafy greens, broccoli, and bell peppers helps control blood sugar levels.

When consumed in moderation, whole grains such as brown rice, quinoa, or whole wheat pasta can supply complex carbs that break down more gradually and avoid sudden spikes in blood sugar. Cooking with heart-healthy fats, such as avocado or olive oil, enhances flavor and facilitates the absorption of fat-soluble vitamins.

Try enhancing the flavor of your food by experimenting with herbs and spices instead of using too much salt.

Legumes like lentils or chickpeas can also be included for extra fiber and plant-based protein, making them a part of a balanced and pancreas-friendly diet.

## DESSERTS AND SNACKS

Making appropriate snack choices can help control blood sugar levels in between meals. Snacking is an essential component of a pancreas-healthy lifestyle. Choose protein-rich and healthy-fat-rich snacks, like yogurt with fresh fruit, a slice of cheese, or a handful of nuts or seeds. These options give you long-lasting energy without sharp spikes in blood sugar.

Moderation is essential when it comes to sweets. Select sweets that use fruit or other natural sweeteners like stevia or monk fruit as an alternative. Utilizing whole grain flour in baking and adding nuts or seeds can improve nutritious content while lowering the effect on blood sugar. Instead of sticking to the tried-and-true fats, try experimenting with recipes that call for healthy fats like avocado or coconut oil.

Choosing foods high in nutrients, ensuring that macronutrients are balanced, and paying attention to portion sizes are all important components of living a pancreas-healthy lifestyle. Developing a tasty and diverse diet guarantees the health of your pancreas and enhances your general well-being.